Amazing Weight Loss Secrets: The Best Ways To Lose Weight Demystified

Positivity Publishers

[Type text]

© Positivity Publishers INC
First Published 2008

ISBN 1453787933

Cover design by Positivity Media

Positivity Publishers INC
P.O. Box 7103
Leawood, Kansas 66207

Printed in the United States of America

1

Copyright

Amazing Weight Loss Secrets: The Best Ways To Lose Weight Demystified

Positivity Publishers

This book WILL help you

to lose weight and will

reshape the way you

think about your body

and yourself.

You will learn about

uplifting tools that can

help you to go further

on your journey to

finally lose weight, keep

Copyright

it off, and to do this with

confidence.

So, why is it so hard for

so many people to lose

weight? Why does it

seem that so many

people go from one fad

diet to the next? Why do

even healthy diets often

challenge your will

power? And why are so

many dieters willing to

sabotage their progress

even after several

pounds of weight loss?

Everyone knows this

basic equation: burn

more calories than you

take in and you lose

weight, right? Well it's

actually not so simple.

The truth is that there is

a missing link in the

journey toward being

free from unwanted fat.

As any person who has

ever struggled with

weight loss knows, there

are many reasons why

losing weight can be

hard. Moreover,

maintaining your
stamina throughout the
weight loss process is
often even more of a
challenge.

There are also many real
physiological conditions
that further complicate
weight loss. A
hypoactive thyroid,

diabetes, a slow

metabolism, and genetic

disposition can all affect

a person's ability to lose

weight.

In addition to these

challenges, many people

struggle with

psychological problems

from childhood and

programmed baggage that can taint their perception of food, diet, exercise, and their self-image.

Some people subconsciously hold on to the unneeded weight as a means of perceived protection against some emotional threat, or an attempt to fill a deep emotional wound.

These emotional problems can lead to a skewed self-perception and a negative body image.

This lack of self-confidence often leads to depression and more overeating, leading individuals to feel a sense of hopelessness and lack of control over one of the most fundamental relationships that exist:

the relationship between

the self and the body.

As this spirals, many

people begin to feel that

who they are is

equivalent to how they

look. Thus when a

person doesn't feel that

he or she looks

adequate or attractive,

this often leads to even

more depression, more

overeating, and less

physical activity. Then

for many people an

overwhelming

helplessness sets in,

and instead of allowing

themselves to feel the

pain of this emotional

distress and to heal

themselves; some people become numb and even more unaware of their choices.

For many, overeating becomes a way of coping and a sort of drug that gives them an initial high and feeling of over satiation; only to be followed by a heavy

feeling of lethargy and

just plain blahh.

Thus the yoyo cycle

continues, creating a

stressful environment

where neither state can

truly be enjoyed.

Eventually the drug

wears off, and people

need more and more

food to feel full.

However, THERE IS

HELP! You should

understand that feeling

miserable after a binge

or yoyo dieting is not the

solution. You can

choose to feel better and

more vibrant; and you

can overcome the

negative beliefs that

once hindered your

progress.

You can regain your

right to a healthier

state.

You must first

understand that weight

loss results from

combining healthy

eating habits with an

active lifestyle, and

applying the secrets that

we will discuss in this

book.

We will show you the

many tools that you can

use to overcome and to

lessen challenges faced

during weight loss. By

using our proven tools

simultaneously, millions

of people worldwide

have already found it

easier to finally lose the

excess weight and make

progress, by starting

right where they are.

They are now free from

unhealthy self-criticism,

and enjoy a happier,

healthier, more relaxed

state. We believe that

you can do it too! When

you apply these tools,

you will find it easier to

become free from

unwanted fat and to

gain mental clarity in

your journey toward

weight loss and
maintenance.

When you succeed at finally losing the weight and maintaining your weight loss, you will regain a sense of focus and control and will achieve a slimmer, healthier, and more enjoyable state of

wellbeing.

First you must start by

understanding that

weight loss is an inside

out process.

In order to keep your

weight off, you MUST

understand this one

true fact:

YOU ARE ALREADY

WHOLE, GOOD, AND

PURE on the spirit level.

You need to realize that

you are fully adequate

just the way you are.

You must know and

appreciate the fact that

you ARE beautiful,

because within your

body is your perfect

spirit.

Realizing this will help

you let go of the two

biggest problems that

people face when trying

to lose weight: Sticking

with a weight loss

program and

maintaining the weight

they've lost.

Why? Because most

people are attracted to

the idea that if they just

change their body, they

will somehow solve their

problems. Thus they go

on a diet thinking that it

will change who they

are.

The truth is that some

of the diets they use are

not even made to

support a lifestyle of

healthy eating.

Thus people get

frustrated by the rigidity

and restrictions and

they just give up. Those

who do stick with a

particular diet soon find

that, once they are slim,

they still have the same

life, and often the same

problems and

challenges.

This does NOT have to

be you. You can lose

weight with these

secrets; and you can

make sure that you

keep the weight off!

First you have to be very

honest with yourself

about the reasons why

you overeat. You can

then address those

issues and finally create

a lifestyle that supports

permanent weight

control.

We will discuss the

reasons why many

people overeat, address

the coping mechanisms

that you need, in order

to avoid these pitfalls,

and finally give you

practical tools that will

help you to develop a

habit of weight control.

These tools are thought

of as "secrets," because

many people have heard

some of these ideas, yet

most people don't know

that these tools must be

used TOGETHER, in

order to ensure weight

loss and weight

management.

Again, remember that

you must practice using

the tools given to you

EVERYTIME you

encounter the challenge

that these tools

overcome.

After you learn the

secrets, we will then

provide a worksheet

which you can complete

to highlight where you

are, what your goals are,

and a plan to help you

achieve those goals.

Now that you

understand that these

secrets are designed to

be interconnected, we

can take a look at the

reasons why many

individuals overeat.

Why You Overeat

Emotional Eating Trigger: Stress and Anxiety

Several emotional states can cause you to overeat. Many people eat during states of excess stress or anxiety. This occurs when a person is faced with a situation by

which he or she feels

threatened. A person

feels a lack of control, so

the individual's fight or

flight response kicks in.

This evolutionary

response normally

ensures survival, by

allowing a person to

attempt to fight the

threat, or to run from

and avoid that threat.

During this time, the

sympathetic nervous

system slows digestion,

in an attempt to

conserve energy and

prepare for fight or

flight.

The parasympathetic nervous system, which works counter to the sympathetic nervous system, regulates calmness, increases digestion, and reduces the fight or flight response. Research shows that people may overeat in times of stress, in order to slow

down the fight or flight

response and thus

activate their

parasympathetic

nervous system.

Thus, when you overeat

when you feel stressed

out, you are actually

intuitively attempting to

calm yourself down by

regulating your body.

Solution to Stress

Eating:

When you feel stress or

anxiety, your response

should be exercise.

When you exercise, you

are actually allowing

your body to combat the

perceived threat in ways

that your body is

designed to. By working

out, you relieve stress

and release endorphins

(powerful hormones that

make you feel good).

This signals to your

body that conditions are

safe, and allows you to

think clearly; so that

you can more effectively

solve the problems that

cause you to feel

stressful.

Trigger: Depression

Not only do some people

overeat when they are

depressed, but

overeating can actually

cause depression. Do
you feel sluggish, tired,
and down all the time?

Feeling depressed every
once in a while is quite
normal; however when
you feel depressed and
apathetic continuously
for more than a few

weeks, you may be

clinically depressed.

Moreover, what you eat

is a likely contributor.

The neurotransmitters

Dopamine and serotonin

regulate mood in the

brain. When the brain

releases serotonin, a

person feels calm and

relaxed.

When dopamine is

released by the brain, a

person feels alert and

focused, more upbeat,

and can think clearly.

When a person eats

healthy foods such as

proteins, dopamine

levels increase.

However, when a person

eats simple

carbohydrates, the body

increases its serotonin

levels. Excess simple

carbohydrate

consumption, as in the

case of overeating, leads

to excess serotonin and

depression.

Moreover, consuming

junk food actually

interferes with the

brain's dopamine

receptors and thus

reduces a person's

ability to feel good.

Then, a person eats
more simple
carbohydrates and
"comfort foods," in an
attempt to feel better.
Unfortunately, the
reason why these foods
are "comforting" is
because they increase
serotonin, which then
continues the cycle of

over-sedation and

eventually leads to

obesity.

Solution to Depressive

Eating:

Eating more raw green

vegetables and protein

will help combat

depressive eating.

Eating complex

carbohydrates, instead

of simple carbohydrates

will also regulate brain

chemistry.

Moreover, when you feel

depressed, you should

try to go out and be

more social, even if you

don't feel like it. This

will eventually elevate

your mood. When you

feel very depressed, just

making sure that you

are doing everyday tasks

like bathing, shaving,

and brushing your hair

will help you to

establish a routine; so

that you can begin to

feel better.

Taking walks and mild

exercise is also

important during

depression and will not

only improve your mood,

allow you to get fresh air

and sunlight, but will

also increase your

metabolism.

Trigger: Self –

Intoxication

While some people

overeat due to

depression, others

actually intentionally

overeat. Individuals

may do so in an attempt

to feel sedated to the

point that they don't feel

their emotions.

Simply stated, food is a

drug. While most

individuals get the

sedative effects of

overeating

unintentionally, self-

intoxicators are unique,

in that they purposefully

overeat in order to cope

with their problems and

become temporarily

drugged.

Solution to Self-Intoxication

If you are a self –

intoxicator, you must

first let go of guilt. You

must forgive yourself of

any perceived

shortcoming, and must

allow yourself to know

that you can solve your

problems WITHOUT

overeating.

You must then find an

alternate activity to

engage in, when you feel

the need to binge. You

may find it helpful to

write down what you are

feeling when you want

to binge.

Then step away and let

the problem fade and

only solutions remain.

The key to overcoming

overeating, especially

binge eating, is that you

need introduce an

ALTERNATE activity,

when you feel the need to overeat. Ideally, that activity should be something healthy you enjoy or some form of exercise.

Trigger: Eating to Fill Emotional Emptiness

Many people overeat because they have

emotional problems that

often date back to

childhood. Often people

feel unloved or

neglected, which creates

a sad emptiness that

they try to fill with food.

The more these feelings

surface, the more people

eat to fill the void.

Solution to Emptiness

Overeating:

Admitting that you have

unmet needs is

important. You can then

allow yourself to grieve

for the loss that you are

trying to fill. Breathe a

sigh of relief and let

yourself know that you

are still worthy, just as

you are. You must be

kind and loving to

yourself.

 You have to become

your biggest fan and tell

yourself encouraging

and constant

affirmations every day.

Once you love and value

yourself, you can then

be in loving

relationships, were you

are treated with value

and appreciation.

Remind yourself several

times daily that you are

wholesome, and that

you did not deserve to

be treated unloving

manner or to be

neglected.

Have faith in your

Higher Power and know

that even when you felt

unloved, deprived,

abused, and neglected;

God loved you and it's

time that you start to

love yourself as well.

Mindless Eating

Trigger: Eating While Distracted

Many people find that they engage in unconscious eating. People often eat while they watch television or at social functions only to find that they didn't even realize what large

amounts of food they

consumed. Moreover,

people often eat on

larger plates, which

allow them to pack on

larger servings of food.

Since the stomach

doesn't sense satiation

or fullness until about

20 -30 minutes after a

person eats, many

individuals have a false

feeling of hunger and

continue to eat, even

when they are actually

full and need to stop

eating.

Also, the illusion that

people get when they

read that a label is "fat-free," makes them more likely to overeat. Many people forget that "fat-free" foods still contain calories, and often those calories are not a great source of the essential nutrition needed in weight control.

Solution to Mindless Eating

If you find that you are eating more food than you thought, start to keep a food diary.

This will anchor you and allow you to get an idea of just how much food you are actually

consuming. Try to focus

on portion size and

always know the

standard portion size for

the foods you eat.

Try to use smaller

plates, because research

shows that when people

eat on smaller plates,

they are less likely to

overfill their plates and

also less likely to

overeat.

Also, AVOID eating

while watching

television, driving, or on

the internet. Assign

areas in your house

where you will eat

(kitchen, dining room,

and patio) and areas

where you do NOT allow
food (bedroom).

Avoid eating alone, and
try to keep track of how
much you eat at social
events. Don't be too
hard on yourself; small
constant steps will lead
to big results.

Creating a Weight Loss Goal That Works For You

Now that you have an idea about why you may be overeating, you can address these issues and develop a weight loss goal.

A healthy weight loss goal involves losing about one to two pounds every week. This can be done by eating healthy, nutrient rich foods; and increasing your activity level in a way that creates a caloric deficiency.

Since 3500 calories
equal one pound, you
will need to reduce
about 3500 to 7000
calories weekly, in order
to lose one to two
pounds a week,
respectfully. This may
seem like a large
amount of calories, but
remember that just by

burning 500 calories every day with simple exercise; you will have already burned off one pound in a week.

If you create another 500 calorie deficiency in your nutrition every day, you can easily lose two pounds every week.

You should also be

monitored by a

professional fitness

expert to ensure that

you are getting enough

to eat, because you will

need to eat more when

you exercise. This is

because exercising

actually raises your

base metabolic rate.

Additionally, your body

needs a minimum

number of calories to

function, without going

into starvation mode.

You can chose any

healthy eating plan and

activity routine that

works best for you; but

speak with your doctor

or nutritionist before

starting any program to

ensure that your

individual needs are

addressed.

Now that you have a

solid plan in mind, we

can address the secrets

that will help you keep

achieve success. While

these secrets are

helpful, in order to be

fully effective, you must

use these strategies

together to yield

astonishing results.

Weight Loss Secrets

Secret #1: **The 80/20 Rule:** Understand that there is no such thing as a diet. You MUST be willing to make a lifestyle change and find foods and cooking styles that will be flexible and that will work for you in different circumstances

and multiple social

scenarios.

The secret is that you

stick to a healthy eating

plan eighty percent of

the time and allow

yourself to have

moderate amounts of

your favorite foods

twenty percent of the

time. So, for example,

you can stick to your

eating plan six days a

week and allow yourself

to have some items that

are not on your plan one

day a week.

Thus, while you might

be on a particular eating

plan or weight

management program;

you still have to make

adjustments for the

times when you are at a

party or visiting relatives

and friends at the

holidays.

You may also want to

designate one day a

week when you allow

yourself to go to a

restaurant or have your

favorite treat.

Flexibility is your best

secret. This will allow

you to enjoy the foods

that others enjoy, as

long as they are

approved by your

doctor, while staying on

your healthy eating plan

at least eighty percent of

the time.

When you use this

secret, you will find it

almost impossible to get

bored. Moreover, you

will lift away layers of

stress and the guilt that

come from cheating on

your diet, just by

applying this secret.

Secret#2: **Water,**

Water, Water!

Sound silly? Well think

again. Hydration is the

friend of weight loss.

When you drink plenty

of water, your

metabolism increases,

your body clears out

toxins, and you can

exercise much longer.

Not only will you have

more endurance, but

studies show that

hydration actually helps

relieve stress and

regulate your mood.

Think about it: how else

do you expect to clear

the waste out of your

system? On the other

hand, if you don't drink

enough water, your

body actually stores

water, leading to water

retention and water

weight gain.

So drink your water, at least 10 8ounce glasses daily and more dependent on your body weight. You can read the book **The Obesity Cure** at

www.freefromfat.org

to get more detail on specific requirements per body weight.

Secret # 3: Instant Craving Control and Appetite Suppression.

As discussed earlier, you want your eating to be flexible so that you can yield maximum results. So how are you going to arm yourself prior to going out to eat or meeting up with

friends and family?

You will be amazed at

this little known secret.

Drink three cups of

water BEFORE you go

out to face any tempting

scenario or whenever

you experience any

craving.

The water will fill you up, make you eat smaller portions, curb your appetite, and will uplift your mood. Not to mention how great you'll feel knowing that you are walking into the situation in full control of your behavior.

Why does this secret

work so well? Because

overweight people have

less stimulation in the

left posterior amygdala,

a part of the brain that

is responsible for

allowing normal weight

individuals to sense that

they are full; overweight

people often tend to eat

more out of a false

feeling of hunger, when

they are actually full.

Thus by drinking three

8oz glasses of water

every time you

experience a craving and

before going out to

social scenes where you

will encounter tempting

foods; you will help

combat false hunger

signals.

Also checkout the

bestselling book **<u>Eat</u>**

<u>Your Way Slim</u> at

www.freefromfat.org

to get an actual list of

recommended foods that

will boost your energy,

help you lose weight and

feel fuller longer, and

are also great snack

ideas.

Secret #4: Sleep The

Fat Off!

One of the best things

you can do to ensure

continuous weight loss

and stable maintenance

is to get at least eight

hours of sleep, and nap

if you need to. Sleeping

helps burn fat, reduce

stress, and overcome

plateaus.

Moreover the key to this

secret goes beyond the

snooze. As detailed in

the book **Clarity in**

Weight Loss at

www.freefromfat.org,

there are various

routines and

affirmations that you

can establish to turn

bedtime into a time that

you can relax and take

yourself closer to your

goal. Soon you will wake

up feeling more relaxed

and in control of your

eating.

Secret #5: Maximize Workouts

Use every step as a workout opportunity. Take a walk for ten or fifteen minutes two or more hours after large meals like dinner. This not only adds up quickly, but will speed up your digestive process as well.

Moreover, try not to eat

for about two hours

before you exercise.

This ensures that your

body is pulling out

stored reserves (such as

fat) instead of just

burning the

carbohydrates and

sugars that you just

consumed in your meal.

Get a pedometer and

notice how many more

steps you take just by

adding this new habit of

walking after meals to

your routine. Try to

work out in increments

so that you can get a

cardiovascular workout
without getting burned-
out.

Also remember that low
intensity workouts
actually burn more fat,
depending on your
baseline. The most
IMPORTANT way to
maximize your

workouts, and ensure

that you actually

workout consistently, is

to couple your workouts

with something fun.

Do you like to shop?

Then strap on your

pedometer and walk

around the mall for an

hour. Measure your

steps and try to increase

your steps as you

discover new shopping

venues. Do you like to

watch Television? Then

purchase a stepper and

take steps while you

watch your favorite

show.

If you are not ready for exercise equipment, just walk up and down the stairs 10 times during each commercial, or walk around your home. The point is that you need to link your activity with hobbies you love and already enjoy. Read **The**

<u>Ultimate Exercise</u>

<u>Motivator</u> at

www.freefromfat.org

for more tools on how to

stay motivated

throughout your

workouts and other

creative workout

activities.

It's also important to

learn your target heart

rate, in order to make

the best of your

workouts. This is

because there is actually

a level at which your

body burns more

calories from your fat

fuel than from

carbohydrates. When

you are at your target

heart rate and maintain

it throughout your

workout, you'll see a

drastic improvement in

your results.

Secret #6: Chew Gum

This is the secret of

secrets! Chewing sugar

free gum will fool your

brain into thinking that

you are eating, will

control your appetite,

and will help you to

control cravings.

As your salivary glands

release saliva, your body

actually begins the

process of digestion. So,

use this secret every

time you get a craving;

and you will not only

have fresh breath, but

also a smaller waist size.

Secret #7: Think

Beyond Will Power

Often, individuals go on

a diet thinking that if

they can just exert a

certain amount of will

power, they will be able

to lose the excess weight

once and for all. Then

when they overindulge

on foods and appear to

have lost their will

power, they feel

remorse, shame, and

guilt. Well, this secret

will enable you to

succeed at your weight

loss goals regardless of

your will power. How?

It's quite simple

actually. You will no

longer depend on mere

"will" to get results. You

will have a certain plan.

The secret is that, you

will chart an eating plan

that ensures your

success even when you

don't feel like adhering

to your diet.

Additionally, you will

take certain steps to

guarantee that you

reach your goals

regardless of setbacks.

The first step to

implementing this secret

is to device an eating

plan that works well for

you. In this book, you

will find sample eating

plans which you can try

to help you get an idea

of possible food choices.

After you have decided

on an eating plan, you

must then take it one

day at a time and judge

your success in daily

increments. If or when

you have a setback

(overeating or binging),

the key to mastering

this secret is that you do

NOT judge yourself

harshly or become

discouraged.

So what will you do

since you are not

allowed to wallow in

self-pity if you get off

track? You are going to

shrug it off and write

down the real issues

that were happening at

the time that you lost

control of your eating.

That's right; you are

going to keep a dairy of

your feelings.

You are going to make a

note of any

circumstances, people,

or ideas that led you to

overeat. If you don't like

to write, then use a

voice or video recorder.

The point is that you

keep a record of your

triggers, so that you can

better understand your

personal motivation for

overeating. This will in

turn strengthen your

will power and increase

your potential for

success.

Also remember that

thinking about

overeating is NOT the

same as actually

indulging in overeating.

So, give yourself for the

times when you stick to

your plan, even if you

feel tempted to overeat.

In addition to a "feeling log," you must also keep a "food log," where you write down your entire daily intake, so that you can review it later. The third part of this secret is that you realize that you DO have power over your food choices and ONLY YOU have the ability to make sound

healthy choices that will

lead you to achieve

weight loss success.

So keep the big picture

in mind, and remember

that you can be slimmer

and healthier, even if

you have a few minor

setbacks in your eating

habits.

 These secrets will work

for you with any weight

loss program and on

any budget. You can

achieve success and you

are already on the way

to achieving your weight

loss goal. But we are

not finished.

Now we will address

your particular needs by

providing a worksheet

that you need to fill out,

to clearly outline your

personal weight loss

goals and map out a

plan to achieve weight

loss success. You will

also find sample eating

plans to help you get

started. But don't stop there.

After you have established a plan, you'll need to reassess your progress on a monthly basis. If you find that you've hit a plateau after several pounds of weight loss, then journal your food

intake and follow the

steps more consistently.

Ask yourself which

trigger is causing you to

overeat, implement the

solution for that trigger

and use each of the

secrets together, every

time you are faced with

a challenge that the

secret resolves.

These strategies have

helped many individuals

lose the excess weight

and keep it off. So, have

confidence and apply

the tools you've just

learned continuously,

consistently, and

confidently until you

reach your weight loss

goals and beyond.

Weight Assessment

Worksheet

1. Why do you want to lose weight? Write a detailed statement about why you want to lose weight.

Weight Assessment

Worksheet

2. When was the last time
   that you were at a
   healthy weight?

Weight Assessment

Worksheet

3. What is your ideal weight
   and what do you think
   will change once you
   reach that weight?

Weight Assessment

Worksheet

4. What was your concept of food when you were growing up, and what role did food play in reward and punishment?

Weight Assessment

Worksheet

5. What would your typical
   day look like once you
   are at your ideal weight?

Weight Assessment

Worksheet

6. What do you eat (include serving sizes) on a typical day.

Weight Assessment

Worksheet

7. Do you often find
   that you look forward
   to eating when no one
   is around?

8. How do you respond to
   stress?

Weight Assessment

Worksheet

9. Do you eat appropriately when in public, only to binge privately?

10. How often do you exercise and for how long?

Weight Assessment

Worksheet

11. How many times a week do you eat fewer than four hours before you go to sleep?

12. Do you often feel guilty or ashamed after eating?

Weight Loss Goals

Worksheet

1. What is your ideal
   weight?

2. How many pounds do
   you plan on losing every
   week?

Weight Loss Goals

Worksheet

3. What activities do you enjoy, and how do you intend on incorporating those activities into your workouts?

4. How many times weekly do you plan to exercise?

Weight Loss Goals

Worksheet

5. How many calories do you plan to burn during your daily exercise routine?

Weight Loss Goals

Worksheet

6. What will be your ultimate exercise motivator (for example, what will you use to get through your workout, even when you don't feel like it)?

Weight Loss Goals

Worksheet

7. What are your favorite healthy foods (think natural whole grains, fruits and vegetables)?

Weight Loss Goals

Worksheet

8. What do you love about yourself most?

Sample Menus

Success Plan A

Breakfast
1 serving of fruit
3-4 ounces of protein
1 (5 gram) fat serving
2 (8 ounce) glass of water

Lunch
3-4 ounces of protein
2 cups of raw (or one cup
cooked) vegetables
3 (8 ounce) glasses of water
1 serving of starch
1(five gram) fat serving

Dinner
4 ounces of lean protein
2 cups raw (or one cup cooked)
vegetables
1 (5 gram) serving of fat
3 (8ounce) glasses of water

Sample Menus

Success Plan B
Breakfast
2 servings of starch
2 (8 ounce) glasses of water
1 cup of dairy
1 serving of fruit

Lunch
2 servings of starch
3 (8 ounce) glasses or water
2 ounces of protein
1 fruit
3-4 servings of vegetables
2 (five gram) servings of fat

Snack
1 serving of fruit
I cup of dairy
1 serving of starch
1 (8 ounce) glass of water
Dinner
2- 3 ounces of protein
2 servings of starch
3 (8ounce) glasses of water
2 (five gram) servings of fat
3 servings of vegetables
1serving of fruit

Sample Menus

Success Plan C
Breakfast
1 serving of starch
1 serving of fruit
1 dairy
2 (8ounce) glasses of water

Lunch
3 (8 ounce) glasses of water
4 ounces of protein
3 (five gram) servings of fat
4 servings of vegetables
1 serving of starch

Snack
1 serving of fruit
2 (8 ounce) glasses of water

Dinner
1 serving of dairy
 4 servings of vegetables
4 ounces of protein
3 (five gram) servings of fat
3 (8 ounce) glasses of water

Sample Menus

Success Plan D
Breakfast
3 (8 ounce) glasses of water
2 servings of starch
1 serving of dairy
1 serving of fruit
2-3 ounces of protein

Lunch
4 ounces of protein
2 servings of fruit
2 servings of vegetables
2 (five gram) servings of fat
3 (8 ounce) glasses of water
1 serving of starch

Snack
1 serving of starch
3 (8 ounce) glasses of water
1 serving of vegetables
Dinner
4-6 ounces of protein
1 serving of starch
1 serving of fruit
2 (five gram) servings of fat
1 (8 ounce) glass of water
2 servings of vegetables

Sample Menus

Success Plan E
Breakfast
2 ounces of protein
1 serving of starch
1 serving of dairy
3 (8 ounce) glasses of water
1 serving of fruit

Lunch
4-5 ounces of protein
1 serving of starch
2 (five gram) servings of fat
3 servings of vegetables
3 (8 ounce) glasses of water

Snack
1 serving of fruit
1serving of vegetables
2 (8 ounce) glasses of water
1 serving of dairy
Dinner
4-5 ounces of protein
4serving of vegetables
2 (five gram) servings of fat
3 (8 ounce) glasses of water
1 serving of fruit

Sample Menus

Serving Measurements and Definitions

Vegetables: Vegetables include all raw green vegetables but not high starch vegetables such as peas and corn. A serving is considered to be 1 cup raw uncooked vegetables or ½ cup cooked vegetables.

Starch: A starch is considered any grain or starchy vegetable. For example pasta, rice, potatoes, couscous, lentils, corn, peas, bread, cereal etc...
One Serving:
1 slice of Bread
4 ounces cooked potatoes
3 ounces cooked rice, peas, corn, millet and other starches
One ounce of cereal

Sample Menus

Serving Measurements and Definitions

Fruit: Fruits that are non-starchy are acceptable, such as oranges, grapes, strawberries, etc... Starchy apples and bananas are classified as starch. One serving is a medium sized fruit or 5-6 ounces of cut fruit or fruit juice, 6 ounces of unsweetened juice, or ½ cup of fruit in its natural juice.

Protein: Proteins are all fish, seafood, meat, poultry, eggs, cheese, tofu, nuts, beans, and peanut butter.
One serving:
2 ounces of soft tofu or one ounce of regular tofu
1 tablespoon of peanut butter
1 egg or 3 egg whites
2 ounces of ricotta or cottage cheese
2 ounces of cooked beans
1 ounce of nuts (almonds, pistachios, peanuts etc...)

Sample Menus

Serving Measurements and Definitions

Measurements:

15 Milliliters = 1 tablespoon = 3 teaspoons

240 Milliliters = 16 tablespoons =1 cup

28.4 grams = 1 ounce

8 fluid ounces = 1 cup

Notes

Notes

Notes